YOGAMINUTE

by

Anita Perry

YogaAnita, LLC
Leominster, MA 01453
www.YogaAnita.com

Book Layout ©2013 BookDesignTemplates.com

Ordering Information:
Quantity sales. Special discounts are available on quantity purchases by corporations, associations, and others. For details, contact the "Special Sales Department" at the address above.

Book Title/ Author Name. —1st ed.
ISBN 978-0-578-13120-7

Contents

If you can breathe, you can do yoga.

—Krishnamachara

ACKNOWLEDGEMENTS

So many people inspired this book. First a big thank you to all the models in the book. They are: Karen Boucher, Karen Cormier, Mary Beth Christianson, Andrew Dorsey, Diane Featherstone, Marlene Feurer, Chris Ferreria, Elisa, Katrina, and Teresa French, Sarah Gibson, Jeff and Maura Lizek, Sankar P. Mitra, Douglas Perkins, Linda Robillard and Karen Wittimer. A special thank you my fellow yogi and photographer, Allison Smith who did all the yoga shots.

Thank you to Chris King, a yogi entrepreneur who just loves to serve, for showing me that this was possible.

Thank you to Diane Featherstone, founder of Frog Pond Yoga Center, my teacher, and gentle goddess of wisdom.

Thank you to my family and friends for their financial and motivational support.

Love to my husband, Charley, and to my two unbelievably creative adult(!) children, Evan and Rebecca.

And lastly, introducing…

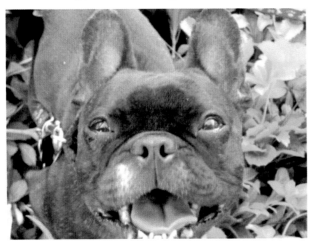

Mocha-The Down Dog

Look for her tips throughout the text!

Introduction

Hello. I know you! You're the busy mom with kids. You need to organize yourself, your children and your household. You're the busy mom with kids who also has a full time job outside of the home as well. Your maneuvers and tactics are worthy of a four star general. You're the full time mom, with a full time job, with a very demanding job. You must coordinate your work responsibilities, schedule time for extra assignments and balance that with your home life as well. I know you. You may be older now. You've been through the Jane Fonda aerobics generation. Your knees aren't what they used to be and frankly either is your bladder. Jumping up and down is not quite your thing. Now you are looking for something different. Something that will help you age gracefully, protect your flexibility and maybe help with balance.

I know you because I am you. I am the busy mom with two children also working a fulltime job outside the home (teaching other people's children). I've also been the PTO officer, band booster, church volunteer, committee member, go to staff person, mentor, and super dedicated, above and beyond employee. I've found something to help in my life and now I'd like to share it with you.

What I've found is yoga. A few years ago when my knees just couldn't take another step aerobics and zumba class, I discovered pilates and then yoga. Soon, I made the decision to become a certified yoga instructor. The time I spent studying to be an instructor was one of the most fulfilling oneof my life. I became inspired by my teacher, a practicing yogi of over 35 years, and tried to soak up as much wisdom as I could, along with poses, Sanskrit, and anato-my. I became friends with the women and men who went on the journey with me all of them coming to the study of yoga from different areas of their lives.

OK, I can see you shaking your head perhaps saying, "**Yes, I know I have to be healthy. Yes, I know I have to exercise. I know it's good for me. But who has the time?**" That's why I have written this for you. It's called <u>YOGAMINUTE.</u> Yes, one minute, sixty seconds. Even a busy person like you can carve out one minute a day. Read on to learn more.

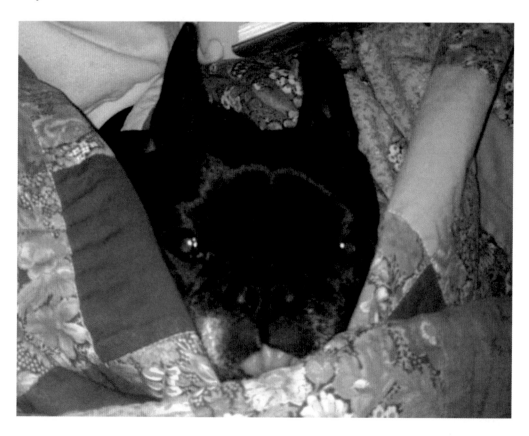

"This is the life! Relaxing!"

CHAPTER ONE

What is Yoga?

Before we get started, you're probably wondering what yoga is all about. All most people know about yoga is the practice or asana part. There are many misconceptions out there about yoga so here are the basics:

Patanjali is an Indian yogi who is considered the Father of Ayurvedic Medicine and the author of the Yoga Sutra. This was written down about 200CE but have course was practiced for many years before that. Yoga originally was only for the elite males. Young boys wishing to be initiated were sent to learn from a teacher. Many of the poses were designed for young, preadolescent, limber boys. (That explains some things, doesn't it!) The Ashtanga refers to the eight limbs of yoga to which every learned yogi aspires. They consist of: Yama, Niyamas, Asana, Pranayama, Pratyahara, Dharana, Dhyana, and Samadhi.

The Eight Limbs

The **Yama** consists of a series of observances for right living. They are:

1. Ahimsa-non-harming
2. Satya-truthfulness
3. Asteya-Non-stealing

4..Brahmacharya-celibacy, clean living
5. Aparigrapha-non-judgement, non-hoarding

The **Niyamas** are personal practices consisting of:

6. Saucha- cleanliness in body and mind
7. Santosha-contentment
8. Tapas-fevor in practice
9. Svadhyaya-introspection and study
10.Ishvarapranidhana-surrender to God

__Asana__ is the series of postures or poses in yoga practice.

__Pranayama__ is composed of two Sanskrit words, prana, life force or vital energy and ayama, to extend or draw out. It is the practice of using the breath and controlling the breath in yoga practice.

__Pratyahara__ is the bridge between, bringing awareness to reside deep within oneself. The goal is to free the senses and rest in inner space.

__Dharana__ starts with concentration, which then merges into meditation.

__Dhyana__ is cultivating meditation, concentration, and removal of obstacles so that the student can achieve Samadhi.

__Samadhi__ is the blissful union, completeness, and enlightenment.

__Samyama__ is the result when Dharana, Dhyana and Samadhi are achieved.

Yoga comes from Sanskrit, which means union and discipline. All genuine yoga is concerned with enlightenment. It attempts to create a state where we are present in every action and movement. Yoga is also to be with the Divine, a power higher and greater than oneself. It's content is universal. In Yoga there is the Cit (consciousness); Buddi, the intellect; Chitta, the mind; Ahamkara, the sense of "I"; and the Manas, the power behind the senses.

Yoga is not a religion, yet it contains universal truths that can be applied to any belief or non-belief system. You do not have to be a vegetarian or super flexible or chant "ohm" for hours on end. Instead yoga is for everyone and everyone can do it.

Regular yoga practice has some great benefits for you and here are just a few:

BODY

> Develops a strong and flexible body
> Increases balance, body awareness, and coordination
> Improves digestion, circulation, and elimination

MIND

> Calms and clears the mind
> Relieves tension and stress
> Promotes thinking and memory
> Reduces stress and anxiety

SPIRIT

> Builds confidence and self-esteem
> Develops discipline and self-control
> Encourages social awareness and responsibility
> Inspires respect for self and others

In my yoga practice, on my website and on my business cards I state: *Calm the mind, stretch the body and invigorate the spirit*. This is because I truly believe that yoga will do these things for you, as they have for many others and myself.

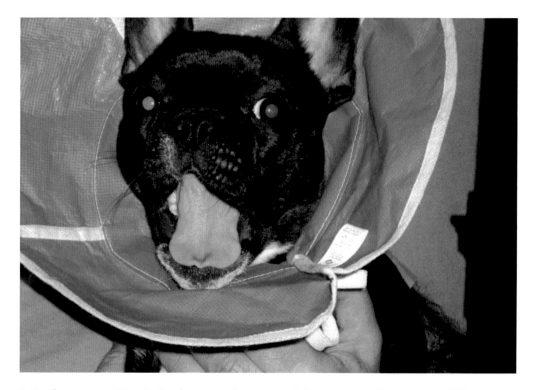

Mocha says, "Isn't it time to do something great for yourself before you have to be in a silly collar like this?"

CHAPTER TWO

How to Use this Book

In a perfect world, you would be able to devote an hour or more, at least three times a week, to your yoga asana practice. But in the real world, there are meetings, deadlines, babysitters, kids activities, committee meetings, another fundraiser to plan or implement, and perhaps costs inhibiting your participation at yoga class. Maybe there's not even a class near you, or you don't know anything about it so you don't feel comfortable enough to go. So as a yoga instructor I would say, try to find a teacher that you really like, bite the bullet and try it out. You'll be hooked once you find the right class for you. As a busy mom and full time teacher, I also say any minute you can take out of your busy day to devote to yoga is a worthwhile minute. You will be rewarded in so many ways. You might notice that your reactions to situations are less intense. You might find yourself smiling a bit more. You might experience more patience with your children and spouse. People might start saying that you look better or there's something new about you.

In this book I am going to group poses and activities together according to their benefits. You will have many to choose from. Flip through the sections first to find the one that speaks to you. There is no need to start with any particular pose or breathing exercise.

Eventually you find your favorites that you will use again and again. Then once you have mastered your favorites, challenge yourself to try something new. I have also included the Sanskrit name because I think it is cool to learn. I will try to be as detailed as I can, but if for some reason you don't understand something, feel free to contact me (aperry@yogaanita.com) or go to my website: www.YogaAnita.com. Many of the poses can be adapted to sitting in a chair if you have a bad back or sore knees. It's not cheating and you still get the same benefits. I am truly blessed to be in a profession where I feel I can make a difference in your life and well-being. Thank you for starting this journey!

CHAPTER THREE

Breathing

Perhaps the easiest place to start is with breathing exercises. After all, you don't even have to think about breathing, unless you happen to have blocked nasal passages or you are prone to asthma or allergic reactions. Most of the time you take it for granted as it is an automatic function. So what if you could use this automatic function to your benefit to help calm the body and relax the nervous system?

Nose Breathing

The first breathing exercise to try is traditional nose breathing. In this exercise, you simply inhale and exhale through the nose. Let's try it now while you are reading:

1.   Let's start with four counts. Inhale through the nose, counting slowly to four.

2.   Hold the breathe inside your body for two counts.

3.   Completely exhale through the nose for four counts.

How easy it that? You've just controlled your breathing! You thought about it (which is called being mindful) and you directed your breath. And though you don't realize it, all these wonderful things are going on inside your body when you do that-like lowering your blood pressure and relaxing some muscles. Now, if you want, you can get fancy with it. Here's how:

1.   Pick an area of your body that needs extra attention. For instance, maybe you've just spent too much time hunched over your desk and your neck and shoulders are killing you. Direct your breath to those areas. Inhale through your nose using four counts. Hold the breath inside for two counts then exhale for four counts. Gradually increase the amount of counts you inhale-hold-exhale.

2.   Direct your breath to your abdomen, your chest, your facial area and then back down again using the same counting system. You can use this series as a wakeup exercise, a mid day refresher, or as an end of the day relaxation.

3.   If you have time and are alone, close your eyes and visualize your breath entering different areas of your body as you inhale-hold-exhale.

4.   Talk to yourself! Add a positive intention as you breathe. As you inhale say to yourself "I am" and as your exhale say to yourself " (your positive intention)" For instance if you feeling stressed, inhale saying to yourself, "I am" and exhale saying to yourself "calm".

You should automatically feel the results of intentional breathing. Repeat as many times as you need to feel completely relaxed

Throat Breathing

Another method of breathing in yoga is called the Ujjayi Breath. With this method, you breathe in through the nose and exhale through the throat, making a sound in the back of the throat. It produces a sound similar to an ocean wave or like Darth Vader in his big, black helmet. Usually this type of breathing is used when doing a strenuous pose or when you need a cleansing breath. Visualize your children tracking mud onto your nice clean kitchen floor that you just spent time sweeping, mopping and polishing and you get the idea. You can also use this breath to warm up the body. I like to incorporate it when doing poses during late Fall and Winter when I feel chilled to the bone. Practice your counting system, gradually increasing the amount of counts for inhalation, holding, and exhalation.

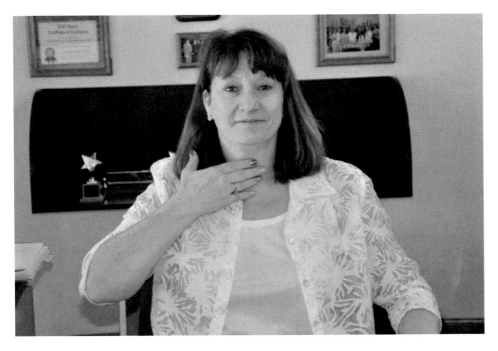

Throat Breathing

Sitali Breathing

Is your boss giving you grief? Has a driver just cut you off or pulled another equally idiotic driving maneuver? Here's the yogic breath for you!

1.   Start by rolling your tongue into a tube. Breathe through this tube and feel the cool, calming air.

2.   Move your tongue to the roof of your mouth. Open the lips and keep the teeth together. (Think insincere, phony smile).

3.   Now exhale through your clenched teeth, with an audible hissing sound. Exhale long and hard getting out all that built up tension and aggravation with your breath. Repeat.

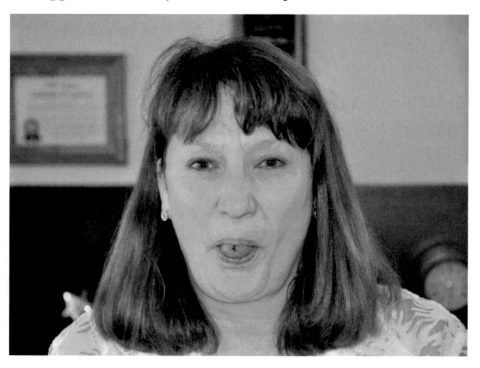

sitali breathing

As you did with the other yogic breaths, gradually increase the amount of counts of your inhalation, holding, and exhalation. Directing your breath with any of the above methods is going to visibly and internally relaxes you, help to lower your blood pressure, and hopefully guide your response to tense situations into a more positive outcome.

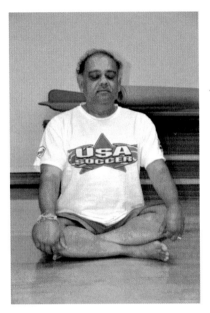

Sitting in easy pose and relaxing can increase your productivity and calm your mind.

CHAPTER FOUR

Neck and Shoulders

Did you know that the average human head weighs about 8-10 pounds? And, as your chiropractor will tell you, every inch that the head moves forward in posture, it increases the weight of the head on the neck by 10 pounds! A forward neck posture of 3 inches increases the weight of the head on the neck by 30 pounds and the pressure put on the muscles increases 6 times. Talk about having the weight of the world on your neck and shoulders!

One of the easiest ways to eliminate this forward neck posture is to reposition your computer screen or car seat so that the neck is aligned. Also, check out how you are sitting on the couch or even relaxing reading a book, using your phone or your tablet. You might have to add a pillow for support. Another cause of forward neck strain is a backpack or purse that is too heavy. Finally, check your pillow. Is it time for a new one?

Now here are some YOGAMINUTES to help relax your neck and shoulders.

Refocus your gaze

This is simply looking somewhere else! So if you are reading, look up and look across the room, down at the floor, to the right or to your left, or, as my second grade students do, look out the window. You are intentionally refocusing your attention. Do a few breaths (see Chapter 3) as you take a visual mini-vacation. Better yet, close your eyes to remove all stimuli. Feel the neck relax, and your shoulders drop away from your ears. Get in the habit of doing this one minute for each thirty minutes you are hunched over the computer or reading.

Ear to Shoulder Stretch

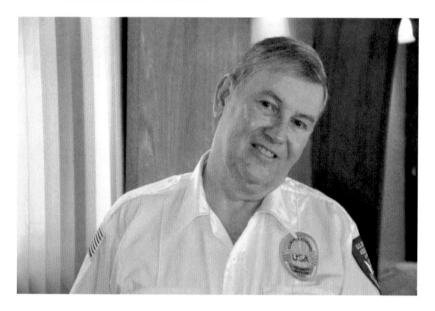

Ear to Shoulder stretch

Sit or stand comfortably. Inhale and let your right ear drop towards the right shoulder. Exhale as you drop the left shoulder down. Inhale and exhale 4-5 times dropping the shoulder further away from the ear. For an extra stretch, cross your right hand across the chest and let it rest on the left shoulder. As you exhale, use the right hand to gently push the shoulder down. Come back to center and repeat on the other side.

Neck and Shoulder Stretch

Sit or stand in a comfortable position. Interlace your fingers and place your hands on the back of your skull. Let your chin drop to your chest. Use the weight of your hands to further lengthen and stretch the neck. Let your elbows point out to the sides. Release the thumbs and let them rest on either side of the neck. Apply slight pressure with your thumbs. Inhale as you extend the neck; exhale so that the chin makes contact with your chest. You decide what pressure is right for you as repeat 4-5 times.

Become a Bubblehead

I'm not talking going blonde here or styling your hair in a retro 1960's style, but making your head light as a feather. Sit or stand comfortably. Close your eyes. Picture a string attached to the top of your head, like a marionette. As you inhale, this string lifts your head away from your shoulders. As you exhale, the string becomes lax and the shoulders come down. Picturing a balloon also helps to "lighten" the mood, relieving more stress and perhaps bringing a smile to your face as well. Repeat 4-5 times.

Shoulder Shrugs

Remember these from aerobic and/or gym class? Inhale as you lift your shoulders towards your ears. Exhale as you push them back down. Add a "Ha" sound to move the breath. Go as fast or as slow as your like. Repeat about 8-10 times.

Shoulder Rolls

Another throw back to aerobics class is shoulder rolls. Inhale as you roll the shoulders towards the ears slowly; exhale as you roll them away. Add a mantra of "relax" as you do so to further release tension. Pause and reverse direction. Start with 4-6 repetitions in each direction.

The Slump

Sit comfortably in a chair, resting your hands on your thighs. Close your eyes. Inhale, growing taller and lengthening the body. As you exhale, start to curl down, starting with your chin on your chest and continuing to lower the head towards the belly button. Let the weight of your skull further extend the neck downwards. Pause. Continue facing downwards, inhale as you curl first towards your center, then coming back up slowly, realigning the spine. Repeat 4-5 times.

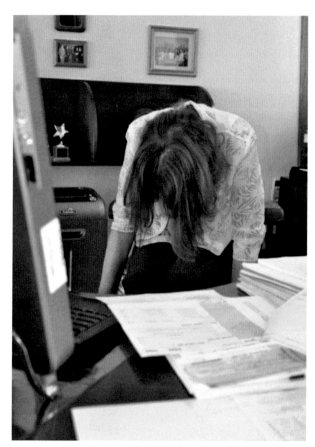

The Slump

CHAPTER FIVE

Standing Stretches

Are you looking for a pose to improve your posture? Do you need extra strength (inner and outer)? Have you been sitting for a long time and need a total body stretch? That's what we will concentrate on next.

Mountain (Tadasana)

Mountain Pose is the basis for all standing poses. It helps you feel grounded and supported. It also helps improve your posture and increases confidence. This is a great one to do before giving a presentation or asking your boss for a raise. Here's how to do it:

1.   Start by standing tall, feet about hip's width apart. Pay attention to your feet and make sure you can feel the balls of your feet under your big toes and little toe and your heel.

2.   Once your feet are grounded forming a strong base, start moving up the body. Internally rotate the knees. Engage your thighs. Bring your belly button back to your spine. Tilt your pelvis down to further lengthen the spine. Lift your chest. Center your head and gaze at a point eye level across the room. Feel the length of your spine from the top of your head to your sacrum, that triangular bony piece at the end of your spine.

Mountain Pose

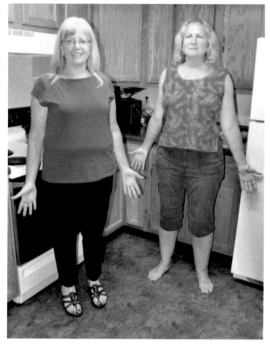

3.   Inhale as your lift your chest; exhale as you drop the shoulders away from the ears. Let your arms remain by your side with fingertips pointing down. Again feel the energy in your fingertips, across your shoulders and down the sides of the body.

4.   Breathe in light and energy; exhale tension and stress. This is also a good time to set an intention, give your self a mantra, or ask for inner guidance.

5.   Your arms can remain by your sides or you can inhale your arms above your head in an H. Some people also like to interlace the fingers except for the pointers and extend the pointer fingers towards the sky. You could also bring the hands together in front of the chest in Prayer position or Anjali Mudra.

6.   When you are ready to release, exhale your arms down by your sides or bring them together in front of your heart.

Crescent Moon (Chandrasana)

You can do this from Mountain pose or on its own. This pose helps to stretch and open the sides of the body. It improves core strength, balance, and concentration. It can also strengthen the ankles and knees, improve circulation and provide energy for the body.

1.   Standing from a standing position, feet hip's width apart, extend the right arm toward the ceiling, left arm down by your side. Feel the length from fingertip to fingertip and as breathe.

2.   Exhale as you start to lean towards the left. Try to keep the armpit open and the bicep close to your ear. If you feel strong and supported, add the left arm extended, bicep by the ear, so that your arms frame your face.

3.   Inhale and exhale as you deepen the stretch. Breathe and hold for 4-8 counts.

4.   Release back to center. Let the arms fall by the side. I like to add a Shoulder Roll before doing the other side. Repeat on the left side.

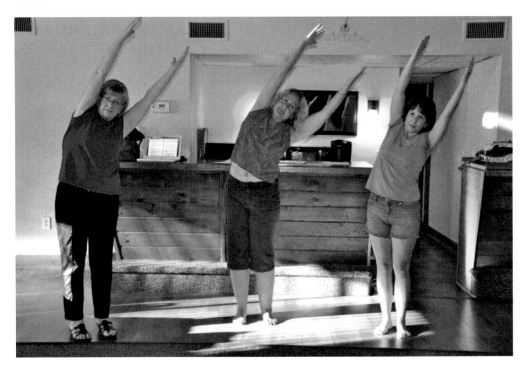

Chandrasana

The Warrior Series (Virabhadrasana)

The Warrior poses help with strength, circulation, balance, and centering. As with Tadasana, they are great to do if your confidence also needs a little boost. Be mindful of your knees in these poses and back off if you feel any strain. Nothing in yoga should ever hurt.

Warrior I (Virabhadrasana I)

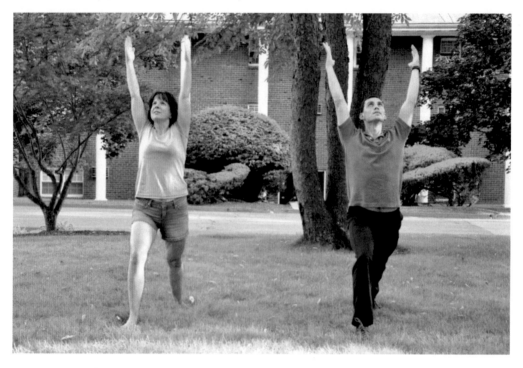

Warrior I

1.   Stand tall. Bring your right foot forward and left leg backbend the right knee so that you are in a high lunge.

2.   Place your hands on your hips. If you can see your elbows in your peripheral vision, then your hips are aligned straight forward. Relax your shoulders down. Bend your right knee no more than 90 degrees. Look down and be sure your can still see your right big toe.

3.   Inhale your arms upward, forming an H, with your palms facing each other.

4.   If you want to go further, lift the head back, and lift the chest towards the ceiling for a baby backbend.

5.   Inhale deeply. Feel your body expand through the chest and sides, and up through your fingertips. Press your feet into the floor and you continue to breathe and expand.

6.   When you are ready, exhale your head back to center first (if looking up), then your arms down by your side. Bring your left foot up to meet your right foot. Pause and repeat on the other side.

Warrior II (Virabhadrasana II)

Warrior II is done sideways on your mat or facing the long edge.

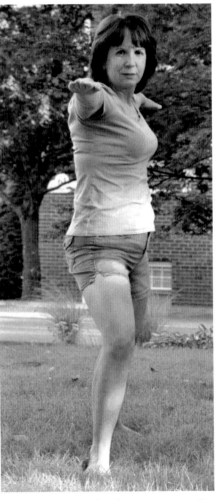

1.   Turn sideways your mat. Open your legs wide. Turn the right foot towards the front of your mat while extending the left foot back. Test your stance by bending the right knee forward, no more than 90 degrees. You should be able to see your right big toe. Adjust wider or shorten as needed to accommodate your body.

2.   When you feel comfortable in your side lunge, place your hands on your hips and again check to see if your hips are level. Can you see your elbows in your peripheral vision?

3.   Sink the hips down toward the floor. Place your hands on top of your shoulders and press them down. Extend your arms out from your shoulders in a long straight line. Turn the palms up.

4.   Feel the stretch in your hips and thighs. Reach the crown of your head up towards the ceiling. Feel the length in your fingertips. Press the chest forward.

5.   As you breathe you can continue to bend the right knee but no more than 90 degrees. Ease off if you feel any stress or pain in the knee joint.

6.   When you are ready to release, bring the arms down by the side. and repeat bending the left knee over the left ankle with the right foot extended out towards the side.

Warrior III (Virabhadrasana III)

Warrior III can be a challenge for balance. You can start by using a wall for support until you feel confident enough to do it on your mat.

1.   From Mountain Pose, step your right leg forward and shift all your weight onto the leg.

2.   Inhale your arms up overhead, biceps by the ears.

3.   Keep the crown of your head long as you start to lift the left leg up towards the back. Try to keep the leg in line with the hip. I find flexing the foot helps.

4.   Look towards the floor as your stretch the entire body from fingertips to the extended left foot.

5.   Inhale and lengthen out before you start to lower the left leg towards the floor as the arms come up towards the ceiling. Lower the arms. Re-center and repeat on the other side.

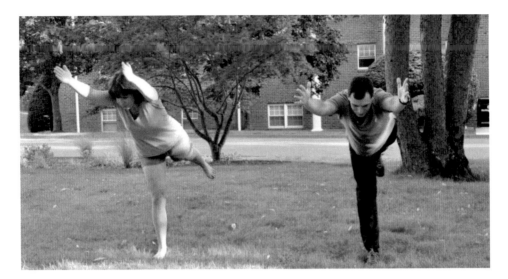

Warrior III

Standing Forward Bend (Uttanasana)

By now you are probably ready to relax your spine, lower back, the backs of your legs and knees. This pose will also increase circulation to the brain area. Try it instead of a coffee break to increase your productivity at work!

Standing Forward Bend

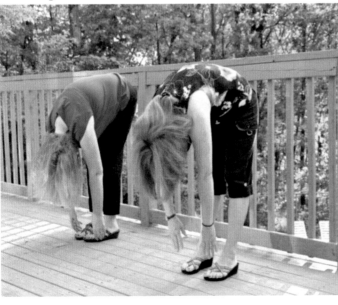

1.   Start by standing tall, feet grounded into the mat. Bring your hands in front of your heart.

2.   Inhale, lifting your arms overhead and then out to the sides as you swan dive forward, bending your knees so that your hands can rest on your mat on

either side of your feet.

3.   Feel the spine lengthen and stretch in opposite directions. Your head is down; eyes open or close (your choice), while the hips start to reach upwards towards the ceiling. Use your breath to straighten your legs as you lift the hips up but keep the head down.

4.   Your intention is to get your nose as close to your knees as possible. Use your breath and lengthen on the inhale and relax your nose towards your thighs on the exhale. Breathe and hold for 4-6 breaths.

5.   When you are finished, be sure your feet are pressed into your mat as you slowly start to come up to a standing position. Keep your eyes looking down towards the mat as you come up, one ver-tebra at a time, so you don't get dizzy.

Goddess Squat (Utkata Konasana)

Time to open the hips, strengthen and tone the lower half. Be mind-ful of your knees in this pose. Ease off if you feel any distress.

1.   Start in a standing position with your feet apart 3-4 feet apart. Turn your feet outwards so that the toes are out and the heels are in.

2.   Inhale as you slowly lower your body, squatting towards the floor. Start with your hands resting on your thighs. Be sure to drop the shoulders back and lift the chest towards the center of the room. Look straight ahead.

3.   If you want, lift the hands from the thighs, raise the arms shoulder height and bend at the elbows with the palms facing each other.

4. Breathe and hold for 4-6 breaths.

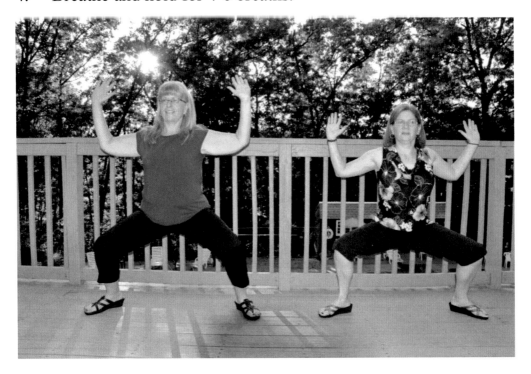

Goddess Squat

CHAPTER SIX

Twists

OK, here come the pretzel moves! First let me tell you why they are good for you and why you should at least try them. In real life you twist all the time and it is good for your spine to do so. As my teacher said to me, "Your spine is your lifeline. You're only as old as your spine." But here's what's going on inside of you when you twist. All of your inner organs become compressed, pushing out blood, toxins, and metabolic wastes. Then when you unwind, fresh blood flows in bringing oxygen and healing. Not only that, you are lubricating the joints, and lengthening the muscles, tendons, ligaments, and fascia (connective tissue). You are also lubricating and maintaining the health of the discs and vertebrae. Use your mat at home or sneak some in at work using a chair or try the standing twists.

Easy Twist

1.   Sit comfortably on your mat or in a chair.

2.   Place your left hand on your right knee. Place your right hand on the floor behind you to act as a kickstand. Inhale and lengthen your spine.

3.   Start to turn towards the right. Initiate the twist underneath the rib cage. Keep your eyes level. Exhale when you have reached your

maximum rotation. Return to center and repeat on the other side.

Easy Twist in a Chair

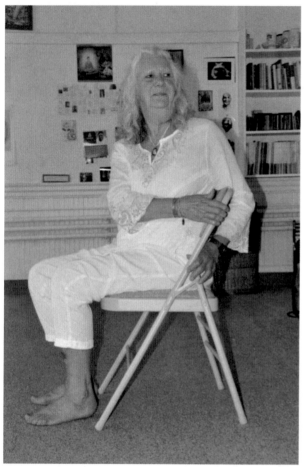

You can try some variations of this twist as well. I like to use a three part breathing method when I twist. Inhale and twist to the side. When you run out of breath, repeat on the same side two more times, using your breath to twist a little further. Give yourself a little challenge to see if you can rotate just a millimeter more each time.

Another variation is to let the chin rest on your chest as you twist. I find it helps to stretch out the neck muscles. You can also let your hands rest on your shoulders as you twist or lift them towards the ceiling. Find the variation that you like best and do at least three on each side of your body.

Half Lord of Fishes (Ardha Matsyendrasana)

Want to do something a little fancier? This is a twist with an extended leg.

1.   Sitting comfortably on your mat or chair, extend your left leg out with your foot flexed. Bring your right knee in towards the chest and cross it over the left leg. Let the foot rest flat on the floor. Press down through the hips and up through the crown to lengthen the spine.

2.   Inhale your right hand up and as you exhale reach the arm around the back with your palm down and your fingers facing the back to keep the back straight. Look over the right shoulder,

3.   Use your breath to deepen the twist. You can also place your left elbow to the outside of the right knee to help you to turn more deeply. Keep the palm up and open. Keep your gaze at eye level.

4.   Inhale to lengthen the spine, exhale to deepen the twist. Challenge yourself to twist a little further each time.

5.   Relax back to center and repeat on the other side.

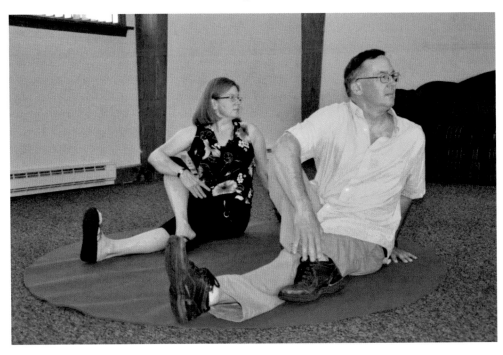

Half Lord of Fishes

Chair Twist (Parivritta Utkatasana) with Variations

Chair Twist

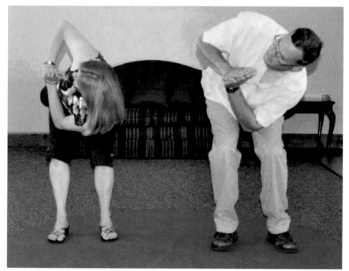

1.   Start in a standing position, with your feet hip's width apart. Bring your hands together in prayer and rest them in front of your heart with your elbows extended out to the side.

2.   Keep the spine long as you start to bend the knees, moving the hips down like you are sitting in a chair. If you feel any pain in the knees, ease off and don't bend too deep.

3.   When you have reached your maximum squat, inhale as you cross the right elbow across the body and let it rest on the outside of the left knee.

4.   Your head is now sideways. You can keep it as is (in neutral) with your eyes looking straight out towards the side of the room. If your neck is bothering you today, you can look down at the floor. If you want to get really fancy, you can extend your arms so that one is pointing up towards the ceiling and the other is resting on the outside of your left ankle. Your head can now follow the lifted arm towards the ceiling.

5.   When you are ready to release, let your head come back to center first, then your arms. Press into your feet as you straighten to upright. Repeat on the other side.

Shiva Twist (Parivrtta Natarajasana)

This is a twist and a balance pose in one!

1.   From Mountain pose, place your hands on your hips. Bend the right knee shifting all your weight to the left leg. Slowly inhale and lift the right knee up as high as you can.

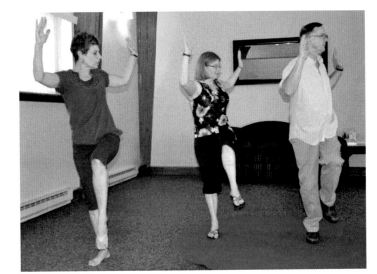

2.   Concentrate on a point to maintain balance. Slowly bring the arms out to your sides with the elbows bent and the palms facing forward.

3.   Keep your legs where they are as you exhale and twist your torso to the right. Quickly find a new focal point for concentration. Keep the left leg straight and strong.

4.   Breathe and hold for 3-6 breaths.

5.   To release: slowly exhale the arms down to your hips and then release the legs back into mountain.

6.   Repeat on the other side.

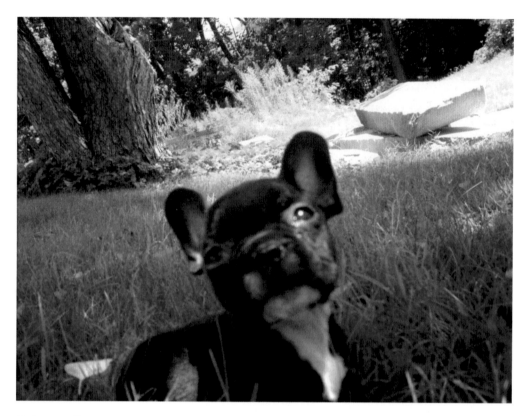

"Never force a twist. Keep breathing throughout and take extra breaths if necessary."

CHAPTER SEVEN

Hip Openers

As we age or during the course of everyday activities, our focus turns to the hips to keep them healthy, stretched, and strong. When I was an expectant mother, I did many of these poses to get my body ready for childbirth (check with your OB first!) These are also great for athletes, particularly skiers, hockey players, runners, dancers, who need the flexibility in their hips to perform to their upmost.

Bound Angle Pose (Baddha Konasana)

1.   From a seated position, bring the bottoms of the feet together, knees bent out to the side. Wrap your fingers around the toes.

2.   Inhale, press the hips down and reach the crown of your head towards the ceiling. Drop your shoulders down. Sometimes it is helpful to elevate the hips by placing a pillow under your buttocks.

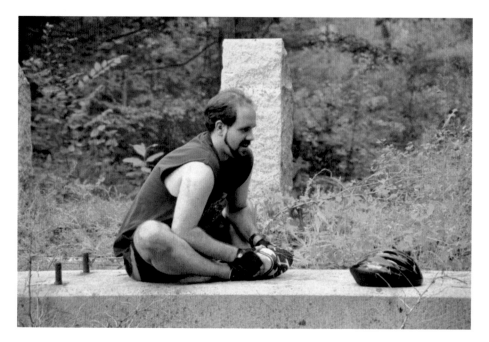

Bound Angle Pose

3.   Breathe as you lengthen the spine upward, lifting the chest. Close your eyes if you wish. Hold for about 4-8 breaths.

4.   You can stay just like this or go for a variation by rounding the back and bringing the forehead towards the toes.

5.   Version three is to extend the feet forward, extend the arms and reach towards your toes. Breathe as you round forward, pulling your forehead towards your toes.

6.   If you are extended forward, inhale as you come back towards center first, and then exhale as you realign the spine to a sitting position.

Balancing Bound Angle Pose (Dandayamna Baddha Konasana)

1.   From a sitting position, bring the bottoms of the feet together with the knees bent out to the sides.

2.   Interlace the fingers around the toes. Breathe the shoulders down and back.

3.   Inhale and slowly lean back so that you are sitting on your sacrum (that small triangular bone at the base of your spine)

4.   Slowly lift the feet off the floor, in line with your heart. Keep your fingers wrapped around the toes. Let your forearms rest near the shins and concentrate on your big toe for balance. Breathe and hold for 4-8 counts.

5.   Release your feet back to the floor when finished.

Half Upright Seated Angle Pose (Ardha Urdha Upavishta Konasana)

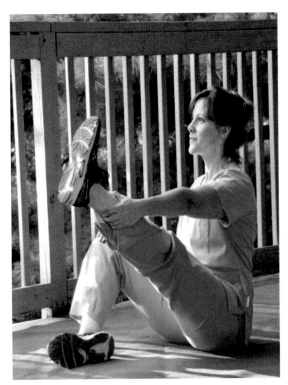

Half Upright Seated Angle Pose

1.   From Bound Angle pose, reach for the big toe of the right foot.

2.   Inhale, as you lift the right leg off the floor, extending through the heel and pressing towards the center of the room.

3.   Try not to lean as you are extending. You can place your left hand on your left ankle for support.

4.   Drop the shoulders

down, lift the chest and breathe 4-6 breaths.

5.   Lower the right left and repeat with the left.

Seated Wide-Angle Pose (Upavistha Konasana)

1.   Start by sitting on your mat with both feet spread as wide as comfortable. The kneecaps and toes should be pointed towards the ceiling.

2.   Inhale your arms up and exhale forward, lowering the palms flat to the floor.

3.   Walk the fingertips forward to deepen the stretch. Keep the eyes looking down to lengthen from the neck creating a nice line of energy from the top of the head to the base of the spine.

4.   Breathe and hold for 4-8 breaths.

5.   To release, walk your hand back into towards the center and then gentle lift to realign the spine back to sitting.

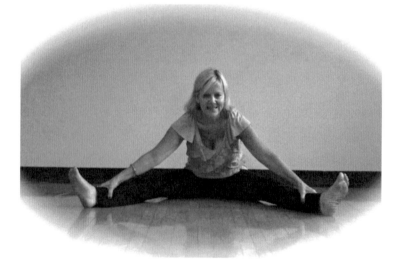

Seated Wide Angle Pose

Upright Seated Angle (Urdha Upavishta Konasana)

This is a bit challenging but give it a try!

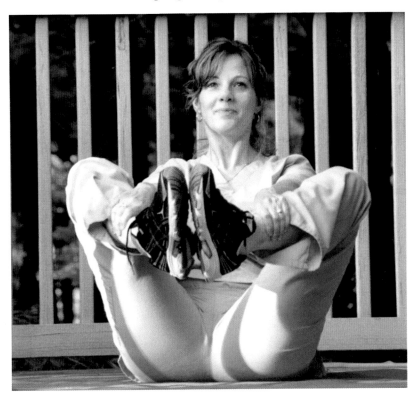

Upright Seated Angle Pose

1.   From Bound Angle Pose, grab the big toes of each foot or hold onto each foot around the instep.

2.   Inhale and lean backwards to lift both heels an inch off the floor. Exhale and straighten the legs.

3.   Concentrate on a point for balance and extend the legs towards the corners of the room. You can keep the knees slightly bent as you are practicing this pose. Breathe and hold for 4-8 breaths.

4.   To release, exhale, bend the knees and bring the bottoms of the feet back together as you lower to the mat.

Supine Bound Angle (Supta Baddha Konasana)

Now you get to lie down!

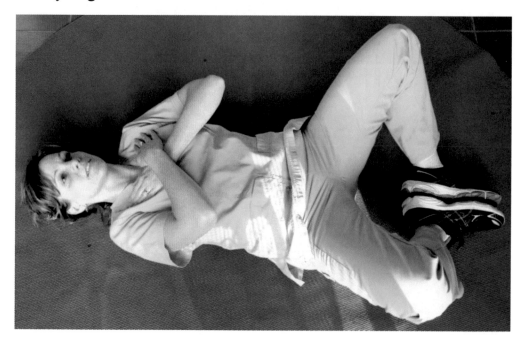

Supine Bound Angle

1.   Lie on your back, bend the knees and bring the bottoms of the feet together. Let the hips open wide but gently to the sides.

2.   Inhale and open your arms so they are resting next to your torso, palm facing up.

3.   Breathe and hold for 4 to 8 breaths.

4.   Exhale as you release and gently straighten the legs.

You can add a bolster or a pillow to support the hips and/or lower back.

Supine Pigeon (Supta Kapotasana)

Another one lying down and one of my favorites before the final resting pose.

Supine Pigeon

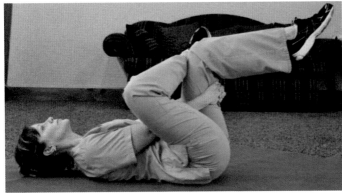

1.   Lie on your back and bring both knees in toward the chest. Keep your head and neck on the mat.

2.   Turn the right knee out to the side and place the right ankle on top of the left thigh.

3.   Reach your hands through the open space between your legs and interlace your hands fingers around the left thigh. Inhale as you gently bring the left thigh in towards your chest. You should feel a nice opening in the hips, thighs, and buttocks.

4.   Breathe and hold for 4-8 breaths. Release back to center and repeat on the left side.

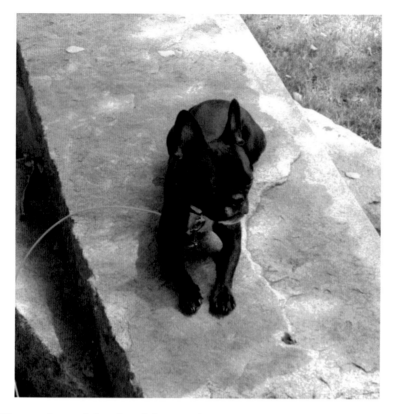

"Keep those hips healthy and strong so you can be pain free as you age. Don't be afraid to use props like yoga blocks, pillows, straps, or bolsters to deepen your stretch."

CHAPTER EIGHT

Back

Your aching back is the second most common complaint in America (the first is headaches). Americans spend about 50 billion dollars a year diagnosing and treating back pain annually and this does not include the costs associated with losing work or going on disability for bad backs. Back pain strikes both men and women equally; usually around the time you are 40. It interferes with our work and pleasure activities, and can precipitate a long spiral of tests, medications, possible surgical care, and health decline. Can yoga help?

Yoga can help you to move off the couch, as being sedentary does not help your body to function optimally. Yoga can stretch and strengthen your muscles and teach you to breathe. Yoga can help with balance, stability, and alignment. Yoga might help you to combat obesity, which increases the weight the poor spine has to manage, putting pressure on discs, thereby elevating the risk of injury and eruption. A recent study at Group Health Research Institute in Seattle, WA linked yoga classes to better back pain management and diminished chronic low back pain including less use of pain medication (http://www.grouphealthresearch.org). Back and knee pain is one the reasons I first came to yoga and I've had great success in remaining strong, limber, and mostly pain free.

If you can devote longer than a few minutes to your back, I recommend Rodney Yee's Yoga for Back Care DVD. Some of the YOGAMINUTE poses mentioned previously will help to lengthen the spine (see standing stretches) and ease back pain as well. Here are a few more.

Mountain Pose (Tadasana) Variations

You learned this pose in Chapter 5: Standing Stretches. Review the basics and then add on these variations.

Variation I Long Stretch

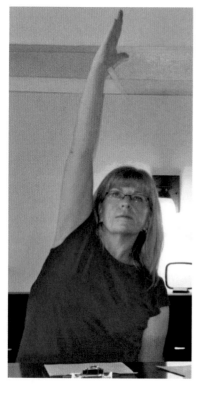

1.   Starting in Mountain Pose, stretch the right arm up towards the ceiling with the left arm down by the side. Feel the length from fingertip to finger tip as you lengthen up on the right and down on the left.

2.   Keep the right bicep by the ear as you continue to reach up and lengthen the body. Breathe and hold for 4-8 counts.

3.   Exhale the right arm down. Roll the shoulder to release tension. Repeat on the other side.

Mountain Long Stretch

Variation II Temple Hands

1.   Stand in Mountain Pose. Stretch both arms overhead, interlacing all of the fingers except for the two pointer fingers. Let the two pointer fingers extend toward the ceiling.

2.   Inhale, roll your shoulders back and open the armpits. Exhale as you lift the chest and reach high overhead. Your eyes can focus straight ahead or lifted to follow your fingers.

3.   Breathe and hold for 4-8 breaths. Release back to your side.

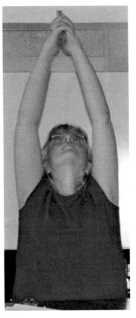

Temple Hands

Variation III Elbow Stretch

Mountain Elbow Stretch

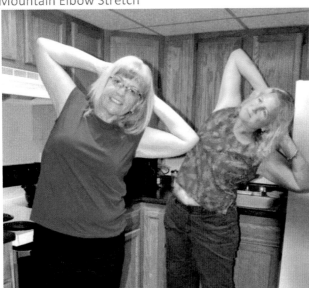

1.   Stand in Mountain Pose. Interlace your fingers and place them at the base of your skull.

2.   Inhale, roll your shoulders back and down. Open the armpits and lift the chest. Extend the elbows out to the side.

3.   Breathe and hold, continuing to lengthen your stretch from elbow to elbow.

4. Release back to your side.

Remember, you can also do these standing backstretches using a wall for support! After you have completed your variations, release the spine by turning side to side, twisting at the waist. Let the arms dangle freely and as you move.

Table Pose

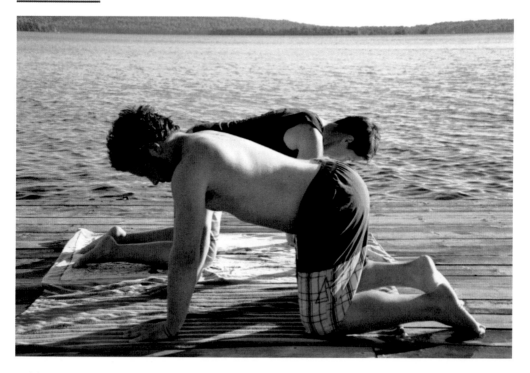

Table Pose

1. Start on your hands and knees. Make sure the knees are hip's width apart and your weight is resting in the palms of your hands, not your wrists.

2. Keep the eyes looking down at your mat. Lengthen through the crown of the head towards the center of the room as you are

simultaneously reaching the tailbone toward the back of the room. Visualize energy running the length of your spine.

3.   Keep you neck long as you breathe.

If your knees hurt in this pose, add a folded blanket or towel to cushion them.

Cat/Cow Stretch (Majariasana)

This is for the middle and upper back and to stretch the shoulders.

Cat/Cow Pose

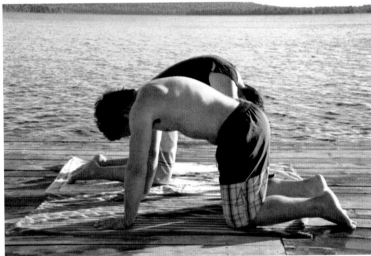

1.   Start in Table pose. Cushion the knees if you'd like. Inhale. As you exhale lift and round the spine. Your belly button is back towards your spine. Your head comes down and your chin should be resting on your chest. Think of a scared cat. Rest here as long as you like.

2.   To continue, inhale as you start to straighten your back, letting your stomach drop towards the floor. The last to come up is your head, eyes looking forward. This is the cow.

3.   Continue to round into cat and straighten into dog for 4-6 rounds.

Downward Facing Dog (Adho Mukha Shvanasana)

This is a classic yoga pose that stretches the back, opens the chest, and builds upper body strength. It is also easy to do it wrong. For this one, I recommend watching a video first or having someone spot you the first few times you do it. Then you can practice on your own.

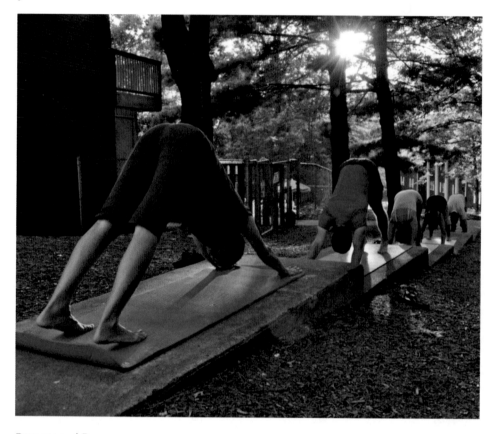

Downward Dog

1. Start in Table Pose. Curl your toes under and start to lift the hips towards the ceiling.

2. Stretch your arms forward and keep your head down. Make sure the weight is in your palms and not your wrists. Keep lifting the hips towards the ceiling as you come up on your toes.

3.   Now you should look like an upside down letter "A". The hips are stretched up towards the ceiling and your head is down. Try opening up the armpits and continue to make micro adjustments until you feel strong and lengthened.

4.   You should still be on the toes. Slowly start to lower the heel to the floor as much or as little as you can, maintaining the length in the spine.

5.   Downward Dog is a relaxation pose. Take at least 5 deep breaths while you are in this pose. With every breath, let the head come closer to the mat as your hips stretch further toward the ceiling.

6.   When you are ready to release, let your knees come to the floor first and then go back into Table.

Downward Dog (Variation I):

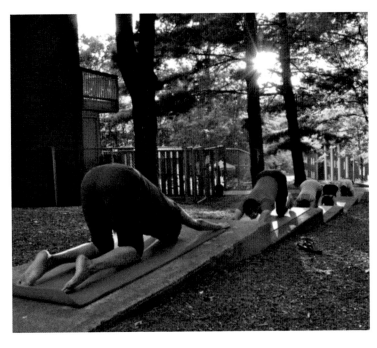

Puppy Dog

If a full Downward Dog is still not feeling good to your body, stay on the knees instead of elevating the hips. This pose is called Puppy (Utthita Svanasana). Keep the arms long and outstretched and you will still get the back benefits you want.

Downward Dog (Variation II):

This is actually another pose called Dolphin (Ardha Pincha Mayurasana). In this pose you let your weight rest on your forearms, instead of the palms.

1.   From Table, lower your forearms to the mat, with your fingers spread wide.

2.   Curl your toes under and start to lift the hips toward the ceiling. Keep your spine long and continue to press through the tailbone.

3.   Start to lower the heels toward the floor, keeping the hips high and head down. Your forward weight is equally distributed on your forearms in the front.

4.   Breathe and hold for 5 counts and release back to Table.

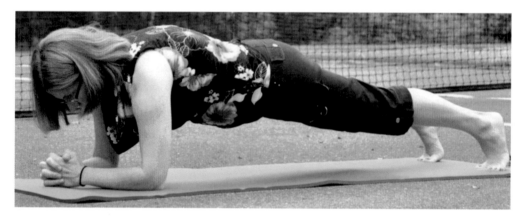

Dolphin

Child Pose (Balasana)

Child's Pose is another resting pose for the body and mind. It helps to stretch the low back and promotes introspection and meditation. This is a common pose to do after an exertion pose. Caution: when I was first learning this pose it bothered my knees. You can use a blanket or towel to cushion them until you are used to it.

Child's Pose

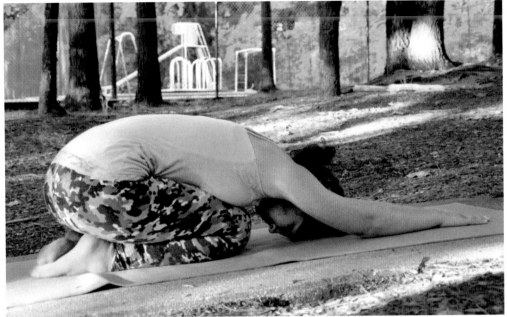

1.   From Table pose, inhale and exhale your hips back so that they are resting on the back of your legs. Your forehead should be touching the floor and your arms outstretched. Some people find it more comfortable to open the knees slightly to the side.

2.   Breathe, slowly and deeply. It's a good time to give yourself a little pep talk, recall an intention you have set for yourself, or just to pause and look inward.

3.   When you are ready to release, push into your arms to balance and support yourself coming to a seated or kneeling position.

Arm Variations: Some people prefer to have their arms by their sides instead of stretched out in front. You can also try wrapping your hands on your heels.

Upward Dog (Urdhva Mukha Svanasana)

Our final pose for this series is Upward Dog. You might recognize it as part of the Sun Salutation Series if you have ever seen or tried it. This pose is known as a counter stretch and will help to improve your posture while alleviating tension built up by slumping forward.

Upward Dog

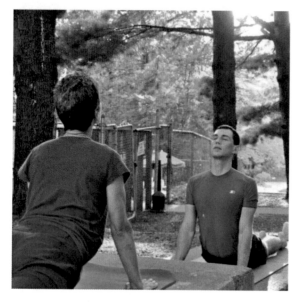

1. Lie on your stomach with your hands an either side of your rib cage, your palms resting on your mat.

2. Stretch your legs back with the tops of your feet touching the mat. Engage your core as you push into your hands, straightening your arms and lifting the torso up. The bends in your elbows are facing each other.

3. Press your tailbone down and feel your hip markers on the mat. Relax the buttocks. Keep the head stable and reaching towards the ceiling, lengthening the neck as well. If you want a challenge, create a little back bend by tipping the head back a little bit. Breathe and hold for 4-6 breaths.

4. Release your body back to the mat.

CHAPTER NINE

Abdominals

Our society is obsessed with flat, six pack abdominal muscles and the clothing to show them off. I'd prefer to think of my middle in a more healthy way. I know that excess accumulation of fat around the middle is not good for my heart. I also know that abdominal muscles that are weak are not going to help me look my best, nor support my lower back when I need them to. So for that reason, I am including some yoga asana poses that will help you to strengthen and perhaps flatten the abdominal area.

Plank (Phalakasana)

Plank

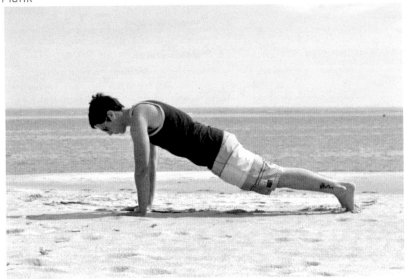

1. Start in a push up position. Your straight arms are a bit forward of your shoulders; palms are

down with your weight centered in the palms. Your fingers are apart and pointed forward.

2.   Be sure your neck is long and your eyes are looking down at your mat. Tuck your tailbone down so there is a nice straight line of energy from your crown to your tailbone.

3.   Breathe and hold for 4-8 breaths.

Sphinx (Salumba Bhujangasana)

sphinx

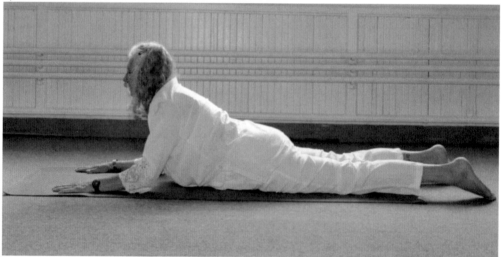

1.   Lie on your belly, with your forearms on the mat. Elbows are under your shoulders and your fingers are apart and pointed forward.

2.   Press the forearms into the floor, inhale and lift the head and chest off the floor. Drop your shoulders down and press the chest forward. Tuck your tailbone down and create a nice line of energy.

3.   Breathe and hold 4-8 breaths.

This pose will engage your core as well as open the chest and align the spine.

One Leg Boat (Eka Pada Navasana)

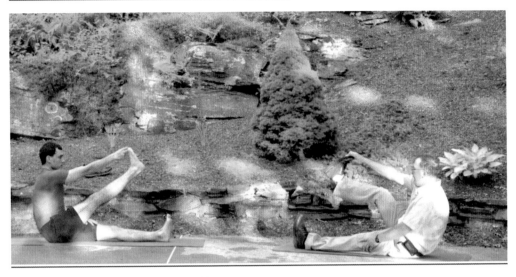

1.   From a seated position, extend your right leg forward. Bend your left knee so that the left foot is pointed towards the right thigh.

2.   Inhale as you lift the right leg a few inches off the mat. Bring the toes back and extend through the heel. Keep your arms extended with the palms facing each other.

3.   Lift your chest and bring the shoulders away from the ears. Your gaze should be on the big right toe.

4.   Breathe and hold 4-6 breaths. Release to the mat and repeat with the other leg.

Upward Boat (Navasana)

This is a challenge pose. You can modify it for yourself by keeping the knees bent or by using a yoga strap.

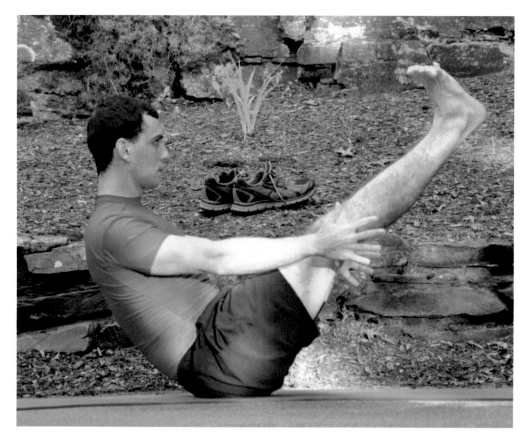

Boat

1.   Start in a seated position with your knees bent and the feet are flat on your mat. Lean back until you feel your sacrum. You may stay here and breathe if you wish.

2.   If you want to go further, slowly start to lift the feet, keeping the knees together and bent 90 degrees.

3.   Again, stay here or start to straighten the legs, kicking out the heels. Your arms should be extended out from the shoulders. Find a focus point as you continue to stretch out the legs from the heels, balancing on your sit bone.

4.   Breathe 4-6 breaths. To come out you can bend the knees back together and slowly bring them to the floor.

Inclined Plane (Purvottanasana)

This backwards incline plane strengthens the whole body, particularly the core muscles.

Inclined Plane

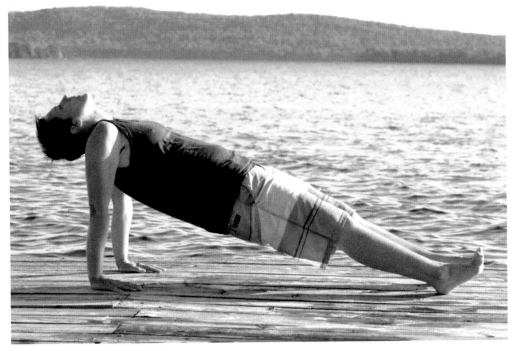

1. Start in Staff pose, sitting straight up with your legs extended straight out on your mat. Lengthen through the crown as you simultaneously push out through your heels.

2. Bring your hand near your hips with the fingertips pointing towards the back. Begin to lean back into your palms.

3. Start to lift the hips up from the mat. Draw your shoulder blades together as you continue to lift. You are trying to get your feet flat on the mat, toes pointed forward as you lift the hips. Gently bring your head back as well if you feel comfortable.

4.   You are now in a reverse plank. Maintaining the same lengthening through the body, engage the core even more as your breathe.

5.   To release slowly exhale the hips back to the mat.

CHAPTER TEN

Relaxation

The best part of doing yoga for me is the relaxation. Granted some of these asanas are not conducive to an office environment but when you are in the right place, the following yoga poses will help to calm the nervous system, help with insomnia, and other ailments that might keep you up at night.

Legs Up the Wall Pose (Viparita Karani)

If you have been sitting for a long time, jet lagged, or extremely fatigued this is the pose for you. It is an inversion pose, which means the pose inverts the typical actions that happen when we sit or stand. It can help relieve tired knees, swollen ankles, and a congested belly. It is useful for menstrual cramps, digestion problems, headaches, and could relieve lower back pain.

1.   Find a blank wall and sit on the floor with your hip right up against the wall. You might want to use a folded blanket as a cushion.

2.   Turn so that your bottom is as flush against the wall as possible. You can shimmy your blanket close to the wall to help. Start with bent knees with the feet flat on the wall.

3.   When you feel you are a close to the wall as possible, extend the legs on the wall. The legs should be slightly open to start with the outside of the ankles on the wall or the soles of the feet touching the wall. Experiment to see what is more comfortable for you. It might take some time to get yourself just right, but it is worth it.

4.   Once you are comfortably situated, extend your arms out by the side with the palms up or resting on your chest. Close your eyes and breathe. You can add an eye pillow or blanket to get as comfortable as you can. Then do nothing!

5.   Try to stay in this pose 3 to 5 minutes to start increasing the amount of time as you get used to being quiet with yourself. To come out, let the legs slide down the wall, bend the knees into the chest, and roll to the side to rest for a few minutes before coming up to a seated position.

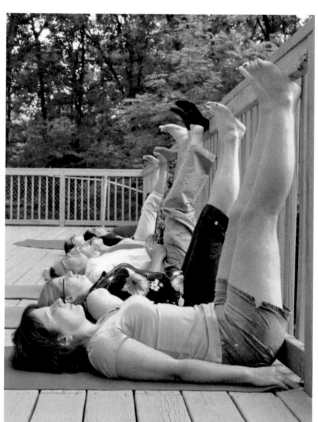

What's great about this pose is that you do not need to be warmed up and you can do it anywhere there is a wall for you. It helps give me mental clarity, especially when I am writing. Don't be surprised if you fall asleep!

Belly Twist (Jathara Parivartanasana) with Variation

Stomach upset or having cramps? Try this series of poses.

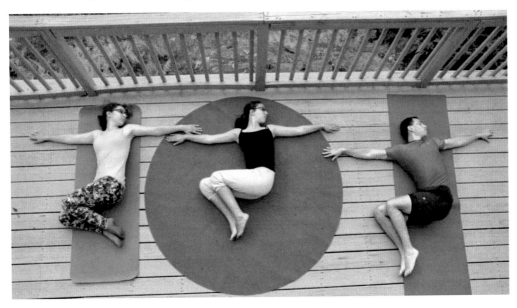

Belly Twist

1.   Lying on your back, bring both knees into the chest, and let them fall to the floor on the right.

2.   Stretch your left arm out to the side and if you want, turn your head to the left to look at your fingertips.

3.   Breathe and hold for 4-8 breaths.

4.   Bring your head back to center. Lift the knees towards the chest and repeat to the other side.

A variation of Belly Twist you can try is to extend the top leg straight out to the side using your opposite hand to stabilize the stretch.

Crocodile (Makarasana)

In nature the crocodile is usually not in a hurry, preferring to laze around the water, floating peacefully. This yoga pose will not only relax your spine, but also reduce tension, alleviate stomach distress, and promote sleep.

1.   Lie on your mat on your stomach. Cross your arms in front letting your forehead rest in the center.

2.   Let your whole body relax into the mat as you breathe. Turn your heels out and let your legs flop to the side. Breathe, pressing the belly into the mat.

3.   When you are ready to release, press your palms into the mat to help you raise your shoulders and upper body to a different position.

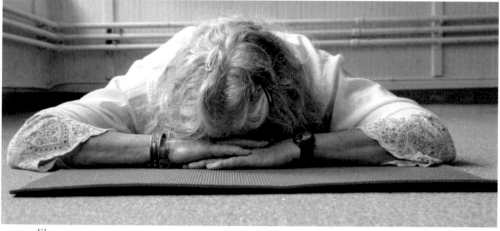

crocodile

Savasana (Corpse Pose)

Even though this looks the easiest, it actually is hard for some people to come to total relaxation and let go. Sometimes the mind is still working when the body is not. Continued practice will help to bring both the mind and body in harmony with each other.

1.   Lie on your back. Close the eyes. Relax the feet and ankles. Let the chin rest on the chest. Your arms are by your side with the palms up or crossed on the chest.

2.   Let your eyes sink back into their sockets or, if you are seeking wisdom, let your gaze rest in the space between your eyebrows, known as the third eye. Soften your tongue; relax the muscles in your face and forehead.

3.   If your mind is racing, try to quiet it by breathing in through the nose, adding a mantra as you do so. For instance as you breathe through the nose say to yourself "I am" and then exhale through the nose saying to yourself "relaxed", "calm", or "peaceful".

Try to stay in Savasana at least 3 to 5 minutes. When it is time to come out, first roll over to your left hand side, pause a minute or two, then use your arms to help boost yourself back to a sitting position.

Some people like adding a bolster under their knees or a blanket to feel totally relaxed.

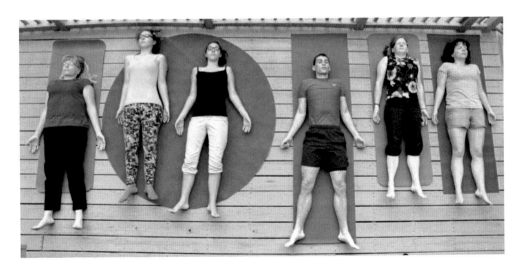

savasana

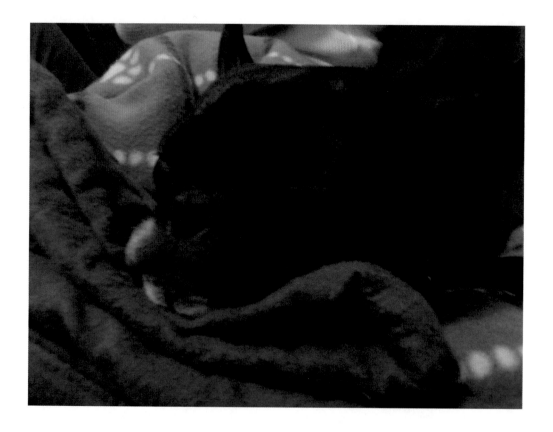

"Savasana is the best"

Conclusion

I'm sure in your readings or through the media you have heard the word "Namaste". This word means *the teacher in me recognizes the teacher in you.* By starting a yoga practice, you have become your own teacher. You will start to recognize when your body, mind, and spirit are out of balance but now you have some tools to help yourself. The benefits of this will be evident in how you feel and in how others react to you.

Do you remember the Seinfeld episode when George decided to change his attitude and enrolled in a self-help program? In it, whenever George was upset he would say to himself, "Serenity now!" Of course because it was a comedy show, George didn't become serene in the least- but you can! All it takes is one minute-YOGAMINUTE-and you can calm your mind, stretch your body, and invigorate your spirit. You deserve it!

So this is the end of the book, but the beginning for you. As I do in my classes, I'll end with these words: May there be peace in your mind, peace in your words, and peace in your heart. **Namaste!**

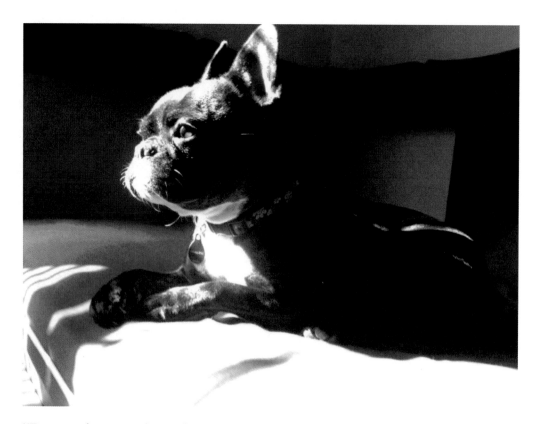

"Remember to take at least one YOGAMINUTE for yourself each day."

Index

ABOUT THE AUTHOR

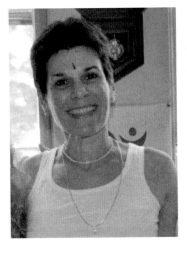

Anita Perry has been in the fitness business since 1978. Though her practice has students from all age groups, her core group is women like herself, in a certain group, going through challenges of self worth, beauty, and relevancy. Ms. Perry was voted Best Yoga and Meditation Instructor by Thumbtack, Inc. 2 years in a row.

Photo by Allison Smith

ABOUT THE PHOTOGRAPHER

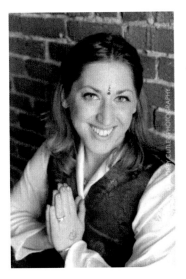

Allison Smith started studying photography at Clark University and has been an avid photographer ever since. Her true love is nature photography, taking wildlife in their natural environment. Allison Smith is a yoga instructor, a Reiki practitioner, thai masseuse, sound healer, milk maid and is founder of Exploga®. Find her at www.exploga.com.

Photo by Audrey Cutler

Made in the USA
Middletown, DE
30 December 2021

57320764R00044